I0707187

SO, YOUR CHILD HAS HEARING LOSS... WHAT NEXT?

M.D. MACLEOD

New research and technology comes out daily that will help towards making hearing loss less debilitating.

COPYRIGHT

TABLE OF CONTENTS

PREFACE

Written to help parents understand their child's hearing loss journey and provide information for them to prepare for the challenges that come with it. This book goes through the general medical information of hearing loss, devices and accessories available for hearing aids and cochlear implants, the steps from diagnosis - getting hearing aids/C.I. - fittings/follow-ups and more, along with helpful tools and tips to help smooth out the process for both you and your child.

INTRODUCTION

The majority of kids with hearing loss are the product of parents with no hearing problem. That implies that the whole family may have a long way to go about learning to live with and support the impairment. Your child could need assistance in one or both ears from hearing aids or cochlear implants. You may discover your child has hearing loss when he's born, or he may be diagnosed later in his childhood. In any case, the most significant thing to do is to get the correct treatment as quickly as could be expected under the circumstances so that you can get your child the assistance he needs to learn, play, and keep up with different children his age. *One very important note:* Hearing loss is mostly thought of by peers as a lack of "volume", however, it is often not as much volume as comprehension that is the issue. Hearing loss does have the need for amplification of sound, but it also needs to address the issue of understanding and translating what they're hearing into usable sound. *For the sake of simplicity and as a reflection of my personal experience as someone with profound hearing loss who utilizes hearing aids, the term "He, His, etc." will be used throughout, however, the content applies to all persons.*

CHAPTER 1

THE INS AND OUTS OF HEARING LOSS

What Are The Causes Of Hearing Loss?

Below are some of the conditions that lead to hearing loss in children:

- Otitis media. This is a middle ear infection that occurs often in young children because the tubes that connect the middle ear to the nose known as the Eustachian tubes aren't fully formed. If left untreated, this condition can result in permanent hearing loss.

- Issues during childbirth. A few children are brought into the world with hearing problems. More often than not, they're attached to a child's genes. On many occasions, it occurs during pregnancy or from pre-birth care.

- Exposure to loud noises: Hearing loss can be caused by environmental damages such as explosions, loud music, fireworks, etc. They can result in permanent damage to hearing loss.

- Illness or injury. Some children can lose their hearing shortly after or during some illnesses. Some of the common illnesses include and not limited to meningitis, encephalitis, measles, chickenpox and the flu, among many others.

Symptoms Of Hearing Loss In Children

Except if your child was diagnosed to have hearing loss during childbirth, you'll likely be the first individual to notice in the event that he experiences difficulty hearing sounds or speech. Below are some early indications of hearing loss in children:

- Failure to react to loud noises
- Not responding to your voice
- Your child is making simple sounds that taper off
- Not understanding directions
- Often ask for the TV or radio to be louder
- Have a fever/ear pain

Treatments

Early hearing loss can influence how a child learns language, which specialists accept begins during the first months of their life. On the off chance that issues get analyzed and treated rapidly, children can manage to escape the issue with language.

Below are some common treatments for hearing loss:

- Watchful waiting (Making sure there is a hearing issue before treatment)
- Medications (Antibiotics) for illness
- Hearing aids
- Implants (Cochlear implants)

Step By Step Instructions To Get Support

Here are a few things that you can do to support your child along with yourself:

- Get educated. There are so many places to get help such as from online along with government and nonprofit groups. They will help you with the latest research that can help guide you in solving this problem.

- Communicate. Get in touch with support groups and join online community chat created mainly for parents whose children are battling with hearing loss.

- Always check in with your child (Within reason). Some kids with hearing loss feel different compared to other children of their age. Be that as it may, early treatment and hearing aids can diminish the odds they'll feel alone.

- Do not remove yourself from your other relationships or the time needed for yourself. Finding support for kids can take a lot of your time. Be that as it may, remember your well-being and of others in your life. Set aside planned time for your partner, connect with friends and participate in activities that you all enjoy.

CHAPTER 2

HEARING AIDS FOR CHILDREN

What Are Hearing Aids?

Hearing aids are small, electronic, battery-operated gadgets that can enhance and affect changes in sound such as volume and pitch. They are utilized by individuals with hearing loss. A hearing aid is accompanied by a microphone that receives sound and converts it to sound waves. It is this sound wave that is converted to electrical signals.

Over 3 million kids in the U.S. have hearing loss and about 1.3 million of them are younger than age 3. More youngsters will lose their hearing later in adolescence. Hearing aids have a lot of benefits such as improving hearing and speech, particularly for children with a kind of hearing loss known as nerve deafness (sensorineural hearing loss). This kind of hearing loss might be brought about by damaged hair cells (sensory receptor cells) in the internal part of the ear, or on the other hand, it can originate from a damaged hearing nerve. The source of the damage will be determined by a medical professional but can be genetics, loud noise, sickness, or in other ways as shown.

Different Types of Hearing Aids

Several factors play huge roles in the type of hearing aid to be recommended for your children. Some of the factors include and aren't limited to physical limitations, health condition, and personal preference among others. There are many types of hearing aids available on the market. New versions are coming into existence on a daily basis. However, there are four major types of hearing aids to consider for your situation:

1. **In-the-ear (ITE) Hearing Aids**

The In-the-ear (ITE) Hearing aids come in plastic cases that fit in the external ear. They are commonly utilized for mild to severe hearing loss. They can be utilized with other specialized hearing gadgets such as the telecoil, a gadget used to improve sound during phone calls. However, their small size can make it difficult to make changes. The only limitation of this device is that it can be damaged by ear wax and drainage and they aren't as powerful as BTE aids.

2. **Behind-the-ear (BTE) Hearing Aids (Most Popular)**

This is what I have worn since I was 3 years old and continue to wear to this day. Unlike ITE, the BTE hearing aids are worn behind the ear. This kind of hearing aid has a wide variety of options and is very versatile. It is connected with a custom-fitted plastic ear mold in the external ear. These hearing aids are commonly used for mild to profound hearing loss and for youthful infants and children. Ineffectively fitted BTE Hearing aids can cause an irritating whistling sound (feedback) in the ear. Be that as it may, a wide range of hearing aids may result in feedback in the event that they are not properly fitted.

3. **Canal Aids**

The canal aids fit directly in the ear canal. They are in 2 styles: In-the-canal (ITC) aid and completely-in-canal (CIC) aid. The canal aids are specially made to fit the size and shape of your child's ear canal. Generally, they are used for mild to moderate hearing loss. The only limitation is that their small size can make them harder to remove and adjust. The problem with these custom-fit hearing aids is that like earmolds for BTE that are replaced as needed by themselves, you must replace the entire aid for Canal type.

4. **Body Aids**

This is quite different from other hearing aids; they are uncommon nowadays but are available. The body aids are hooked onto a belt or pocket and connected to the ear with a wire. They are frequently utilized when a child has very profound hearing loss and when different kinds of hearing aids have failed to help with their situation.

Who Are The Candidates For Hearing Aids?

Most kids with hearing loss that have been found to benefit from hearing aids are the right candidate for these devices. Many factors play a large role in the type of hearing aid that should be used and they are:

- The shape of the outer ear. There are different shapes of the ear; Behind-the-ear hearing aids cannot work for ears with an abnormal shape.
- Depth or length of depression near the ear canal. Some ears are shallow and due to this; they are not the best fit for in-the-ear hearing aids.
- The type and severity of hearing loss
- The child's capacity to take in and out hearing aids
- The measure of earwax buildup

- Drainage: some ears require drainage and as a result of this, they are most likely to be unable to utilize certain hearing aid models.

How to Know if Your Child Needs a Hearing Aid or Cochlear Implant

Many of the kids with hearing loss benefit greatly from hearing aids, but on the other hand, some of them will do better with a cochlear implant. The audiologist and other hearing experts will decide if your child is a suitable candidate for hearing aids or cochlear implant and this depend largely on the type and severity of the hearing loss, and also the structure and shape of the outer ear.

Hearing loss commonly occurs at an early stage of life in very young kids, the use of hearing aids starts at the initial stage and at a later time, when the kid is growing older, the cochlear implant becomes the next available option. A kid with hearing loss will have continuous hearing tests; this is done to carefully track hearing ability and the benefits that have been achieved with the use of the device.

Where to Purchase a Hearing Aid

A medical test is performed before purchasing a hearing aid. Here are some of the places where you can purchase a hearing aid for your kids;

- An audiologist. This is a pro that can evaluate and oversee the hearing and balance issues. You might be referred to an audiologist by your kid's ear, nose, and throat specialist (ENT) or the audiologist may work in the same office.
- An independent company.

Styles and prices differ enormously based on type, power, and capabilities. Carry out a thorough research on both hearing aids and the organizations that sell them. Take note of these questions when buying hearing aids:

- Can my child's hearing loss be improved with the medicinal or surgical treatment approach?
- Which design will work best for my child's type of hearing loss?
- Will my child be able to test the Hearing aids for a specific time before buying?
- What is the cost of hearing aids? On the chance that cash is an issue, are there offices that can help cover the cost?

- Is there any warranty that follows the hearing aids and what does the warranty cover?

- Could my child's audiologist or otolaryngologist make changes and repairs?

- Will some other assistive devices be utilized with the hearing aids?

Wearing Hearing Aids

As soon as the hearing aids have been fitted for the affected ears, it is advisable that your child should start to out on the hearing aid slowly. Note that hearing aids do not restore normal hearing, because of this, it might require a large amount of time to become acclimated to the various sounds transmitted by the device. Below are some helpful tips you can follow as soon as your child is preparing to put on hearing aids:

- It's wise to talk about the hearing aid to your child and show them how it will be of help to them. Allow your child to ask questions about things they would like to know about the device.

- Be patient and give your child time to become accustomed to the hearing aid and the sound it provides.

- Begin using the hearing aid in calm areas and gradually move to louder, busier locations.

- Carry out some tests to see where the hearing aid works best to grow their comfort level with them.

- Track any worries or concerns that you or your child have. Bring this to your child's subsequent examination.

How To Take Good Care Of Hearing Aids

Hearing aids need to be kept dry. Cleaning techniques differ and this has to do with the style and shape of the device. Some other care tips are listed below:

- Keep the hearing aids from extreme heat or cold.

- Batteries should be replaced frequently, approximately every 1 to about fourteen days.

- Try not to use hairspray or other products when the hearing aid is in the way.

- Make sure the tubes (where required) are changed, as well as microphone filters, as these common issues take away the effectiveness of the hearing aid.

The Importance of Hearing Aids for Your Child

In the event that an audiologist prescribes hearing aids for your child, it's significant that the person wears them constantly, particularly if the child is very young. Below are some of the reasons:

- Starting from birth to three years, children's brains are in a time of quick learning. Consistent sound input is very important for the formation of brain pathways for hearing and language development.

- Early listening and communication play a huge role in the development of language. In any case, when first learning a language, we can't actually "teach" it to kids in the manner in which one would train a school subject. Rather, language is gathered from daily experiences. Children learn words and communication including grammar and language structure by being exposed to language constantly. For kids battling with hearing loss, this coincidental learning should be enhanced by speech and language treatment that pays much attention to this auditory input.

- Steady input is additionally significant for newborn babies, children, and toddlers in building a strong relationship with their parents. The outcome of this is the building of trust and allows for the feeling of a foreseeable and dependable world.

- Hearing aids can be principally useful for kids because their young brains are in a time of rapid development. Sound input is hugely important as it improves the development of speech and cognitive functions.

CHAPTER 3

COCHLEAR IMPLANTS FOR CHILDREN

This chapter is brief as it is a surgical procedure that is different for everyone and is intended to give the overall picture of its benefits and drawbacks. As a child of someone with a Cochlear implant, it does amazing things, if you put in the time and dedication required to succeed.

What Is A Cochlear Implant?

A cochlear implant is a small, complex electronic device that can help a person who is profoundly deaf or extremely hard-of-hearing get a sense of sound. The implant consists of an external portion behind the ear and a second portion which is placed by the surgical process under the skin. An implant is made of the following parts:

- A microphone that takes sound from the surroundings.
- A speech processing machine, choosing and organizing sounds that the microphone picks up.
- A transmitter and receiver/stimulator, which receives and translates signals from the speech processor into electrical impulses.

- An electrode array, which is a group of electrodes that collect the stimulator impulses and send them to various regions of the auditory nerve.

The implant does not return hearing to normal. Rather, it can provide a deaf or hard-of-hearing person with a valuable sound representation in the community and offer great help to him or her in other to understand speech.

How Does a Cochlear Implant Work?

A cochlear implant is quite distinct from a hearing aid. Hearing aids enhance sounds so that impaired ears can hear them. Cochlear implants bypass damaged parts of the ear and activate the auditory nerve directly. Implant-generated signals are transmitted to the brain via the auditory nerve which recognizes the signals as sound. Hearing through a cochlear implant varies from hearing naturally and takes time to learn or relearn. This helps a lot of people to hear warning signals, understand certain sounds in the area, and have a better understanding of speech in person or over the phone.

Who Is a Suitable Candidate for Cochlear Implants?

Cochlear implants can be fitted to children and adults who are deaf or extremely hard-of-hearing. As of December 2012, there were around 324,200 installed registered devices worldwide. Around 58,000 devices were implanted in adults in the United States, and 38,000 in infants. (Estimates are given by the US Food and Drug Administration [FDA] as stated by cochlear implant manufacturers.)

In the mid-1980s, the FDA first approved cochlear implants to treat adult hearing loss. Cochlear implants have been FDA-approved since 2000 for use in eligible children starting at age 12. Using a cochlear implant while young exposes them to sounds during an optimal period to develop speech and language skills for young children who are deaf or severely hard-of-hearing. Evidence has shown that when these kids undergo a cochlear implant followed by intensive therapy before they are 18 months of age, they are better able to hear, understand sound and music, and speak than their peers when they are older to receive implants. Research has also shown that qualifying children who obtain a cochlear implant before the age of 18 months gain language skills at a rate comparable to normal-hearing children, and many are effective in traditional classrooms.

Cochlear implants can also help certain people who have lost all or most of their hearing later in life. We learn to associate the implant's signals with the sounds we know, including speech, without needing any visual cues such as those given by lipreading or sign language.

How Does One Get A Cochlear Implant?

Using a cochlear implant involves both a surgical procedure and intensive rehabilitation to learn or relearn the hearing senses. This process is drastically different for each person undergoing the procedure and training. The decision to accept an implant will require consultations with medical specialists, including a cochlear implant surgeon with experience. It can be an expensive process. A person's health insurance, for example, can cover the costs but not always. For a variety of personal reasons, other people may choose not to have a cochlear implant. Surgical implants are almost always safe, although complications are a risk factor, as is the case with any type of operation. The factor is learning to perceive the sounds an implant makes. It takes time and practice for that process. Speaking-language pathologists and audiologists often participate in this learning process. Some training includes speech, television, audiobooks, music, etc. All of these considerations need to be weighed before implantation.

CHAPTER 4

THE HEARING AID FITTING PROCESS

Taking Ear Impressions

The initial step for fitting a hearing aid is usually to take impressions of the external ear canals. These must be taken to guarantee that the earmolds for your child's hearing aids fit properly. This is done by a hearing professional by placing a cotton or foam dam deep down into the ear canal after which it will carefully fill the canal with the impression material. To ensure all the ear structures are well represented, the impression material will fill the whole outer ear. The material takes a couple of minutes to set, so guardians/parents are often asked to hold the baby or child to keep curious hands out of the way.

Earmolds are made available in different colors; this gives a parent the choice to select a different color for each ear to make it easy to quickly determine that particular earmold that fits the ear, this is uncommon but available.

There will be a periodic need for the earmold in the future as the child grows older giving room for color change and desire. The mailing out of the ear impressions is done by the audiologist and in some cases; it may take up to two weeks to receive the custom earmolds order.

Step By Step Instructions To Fit The Hearing Aids
During your meeting with an audiologist, they will ensure the earmolds fit your child's ears appropriately and program the hearing aids for your child's hearing loss. At the point when the hearing aids are programmed and activated for the very first time, your child will start to hear new sounds immediately. Newborn children will, in general, have a prompt response to mother or father's voice, turning their head with enthusiasm toward the parent who currently makes a sound. After the initial programming and activation, the audiologist will do some sound tests to ensure that delicate sounds are sufficiently loud, normal sounds are comfortable and loud sounds are considered not too loud by the user.

The consultation expert will likewise invest a lot of time in showing you how to place and remove the hearing aids, how to connect and disconnect the earmold from the hearing aid and you will also be shown ways to identify and differentiate between the right and left aids (Blue on left HA, Red on right HA). You will figure out how to turn them on and off, how to do a listening check to ensure they're working and how to remove and replace the batteries. You will also learn how to keep the portable hearing aids clean and how to store them each night.

Follow-Up Appointments

The fact is that it will take some time before your child becomes used to the new sounds they perceive. Speech and language treatment will support the newborn child or kid to catch up to same-age peers and ensure achievements for speech, language and hearing are being met. It is also important to schedule a follow-up appointment with your audiologist. This is done to monitor the hearing ability of your child. Follow-up hearing tests will help evaluate hearing capacity across certain pitches and adjust the hearing aids effectively as required.

A decent working relationship with your child's hearing care team is fundamental! Follow-up visits are critical to check the hearing aids and your child's advancement with them through hearing tests and evaluations.

The follow-up visits will monitor the capacity and fitting of the hearing devices. Children's ear canals grow and develop rapidly which can create sound leakage that can cause the hearing aids to produce feedback. There may be a need to replace the earmold extremely often, this is applicable to developing babies and where weight fluctuates in kids or adults, the number used as a guide is with every 5lbs in older kids and adults, and constantly as a young baby or child is growing and developing very quickly.

CHAPTER 5

HEARING AID TOOLS & TIPS FOR PARENTS

TIPS

Lip Reading / Sign Language

This is probably one of the most beneficial things that you will be able to teach your child. It is also something that they will develop naturally as they try to listen to speech, their brain will automatically link the same movements to the sounds they are trying to interpret. For kids that can hear volume but struggle with comprehension, this is huge.

Keeping Them On

Hearing aids only function while your child is wearing them. It's not always easy, young kids might just take them out, while older kids might not like them or refuse to wear them. On the off chance that your child consistently pulls on the hearing aids or his ears, this could be attributed to discomfort from a poorly fitting earmold. When this happens, make sure that you see your child's audiologist as soon as possible to see whether it's an ideal opportunity to get another pair of earmolds made.

It very well may be hard to keep hearing aids on your child, particularly children who have not worn them since the early stages. On the off chance that your child opposes the use of hearing aids or regularly pulls them off, there are a few different ways to make hearing aids more comfortable for your kids:

- Put the hearing aids on your child when both of you are engaged in fun and playful activity, at this period, your child will be less interested in pulling them out or off.

- Attempt a soft headband that you can secure over the hearing aids, however, ensure that the microphone isn't covered.

- Make use of special clips in other to keep hearing aids attached to your child's clothes.

- Lengthen how long he'll wear them all day long until he has them on for the entirety.

- Teach your young child that only adults put in or take out the aids.

- It may be that your child wants colored earmolds or aids. These may be something he wants to wear than simple earmolds.

Your audiologist will assist in finding the best way to keep your child's hearing aids where they belong.

A Hearing Aid Routine

It is smart to build up a schedule every day for putting your child's hearing aids on and taking them off. When you put their hearing aids in, ensure it is a positive time for them, this is done to build a positive relationship with them. At the point when your curious child removes the hearing aids, ensure that you are consistent and gentle in putting it back, this is helpful because your child will be able to know that's where they belong. At night, you would benefit by having a hearing aid box, or dryer next to the bed that the hearing devices go into each night.

Daily Checks

It is important for you to check your child's hearing aids on a daily basis, mostly when your children are too young to tell if there is any problem. It is a good idea to do a listening check, make sure that the battery is working and check the hearing aids in case there is the presence of debris and moisture. Keep in mind, on the off chance that you can't hear sounds amplified through the hearing aids when they're at your ear, your little one won't be able to hear through it, either.

Safety

When you are selecting a hearing aid for your infants and kids, ensure that you go for hearing aids that have secure battery doors this will stop your kids from getting out the batteries of the devices. As we all know, kids derive a lot of pleasure in putting things in their mouths, as a result of this make sure that the batteries are kept away from the reach of your kids until they are old enough to be trusted with them.

The correct hearing aids can improve things significantly for your child's social, educational and communication development. Work with your child's audiologist, doctor and educational support system to take advantage of the experience.

Situational Awareness

This is one of the areas that is very important to teach to your child with hearing loss. They won't be able to rely on their hearing to alert them of dangers such as traffic, animals, etc. and need to be taught to stay aware and use their eyes to know where they are and what is going on around them at all times.

Social Aspects and How to Make It Easier on You

Educate your child on the hearing aids and the part they play to help him hear effectively in daily life. This is also important so when other kids are asking about them, they know what to say, proudly, instead of getting upset.

Accept the hearing loss, it will make it easier on both of you from the start. Think about talking to the school and suggest a class discussion regarding hearing aids and their function for millions of people worldwide, show students that they are no different.

Remember and tell your child, hearing aids are no different than glasses to help people see, they help you hear.

Maintenance and Hygiene

Go over hearing aid operation with your child often until they know it well, including, how to change batteries (depending on age), how to keep them clean, how to adjust volume and turn on/off, how to change modes (FM, normal, directional)

Check and clean hearing aids each day. Clean earwax from earmolds, check tubes for cracks and pliability, get "Tune-ups" at the audiologist (Filters, batteries, tubes).

Keep extra batteries/filters with you and at the school, store batteries at room temperature (not the fridge), and change filters often as moisture makes them plug up.

Find The Best Hearing Aid For Your Child

It is important to note that not every aids works well for every child. As mentioned above, it is the duty of the audiologist to find the best aids for your child. The audiologist will reveal to you what your child should do during the day and what he needs. They also come in many colors and styles for the child to choose, making it easier for them to wear.

At home and school, your child may be able to use hearing aids paired with hearing assistive technology systems. Therefore, your child's aids should have features that work in along with these systems, such as FM systems, Bluetooth, etc. (Discussed later).

The best type of hearing aid for your child depends on his specific needs. The most common one is the behind-the-ear or BTE and this is because of the following reasons;

- it can connect to various earmold types
- this type is easy to replace as your child develops
- it is very easy to handle and clean
- this device easily allows you to adjust the aid
- it works with a wide range of hearing loss

- it can incorporate features that connect with other systems

In-the-ear, or ITE, styles are increasingly popular for grown-ups and older kids with less severe hearing loss.

Hearing Aid Technology

Another thing to think about when choosing the best hearing aid for your child is the technology and capabilities that they have. New advancements can be used to greatly advantage your child in educational and social situations. This means that through the use of technology in the hearing aid, often used along with a component in the home or classroom, helps them hear speech and media on a much greater scale. Some of this technology includes:

Bluetooth – This allows the hearing aids to connect to Bluetooth microphones or transmitters that send the signal directly into the child's hearing aids, like if he was wearing headphones. This can be used via a microphone that the speaker wears, or a transmitter hooked into a television sending the audio directly to the hearing aids, bypassing all interference between the hearing aids and audio source.

FM Systems: This is an older technology where a speaker wears a transmitter with a microphone around their neck and the student wears a receiver around their neck. The audio is received through the hearing aid in ways of a "boot" which is connected to the bottom of the hearing aid.

Bluetooth has more capabilities but uses more battery power, and sometimes has connectivity issues. The FM system is tried and true but has limited functionality beyond person to person conversation.

Overall, there are many reasons why you should consider hearing aids with the technology to help out with daily interactions including school, home, recreation, and entertainment.

TOOLS (Available at audiologist or online)
Hearing Aid Lanyards
These lanyards have a loop that goes around the hearing aid and attaches to your child's shirt, this keeps them from being lost in the event they fall out (and they will).

Hearing Aid Dryers

Hearing aid dryers take the humidity out of the hearing aid's electronics and filters to keep them working effectively and are there in case of accidental spills etc.

These dryers come in either conventional versions or electric versions.

Conventional dryers are a container that uses pellets that change color when they are ready to be used or need to be recharged for use. They are recharged by removing the pellets and putting them in the oven on a baking sheet until they all change color.

Electric dryers are used for the same thing, but usually operate using U.V. rays and heat, cleansing the aid and removing moisture at the same time. These units are quite a bit more expensive but are easy to use and just get plugged into a regular wall electrical socket for use.

Note: Take the earmolds off before inserting H.A. into a dryer.

Bluetooth Devices

These are the devices that work along with a Bluetooth equipped hearing aid. Some popular options include the Phonak ComPilot and the Rogers devices.

Both systems (and the others available) have different operating procedures and connectivity directions, but they are both capable of working with hearing aids. Your audiologist will be able to help you choose a good combination.

Hearing Aid Covers

Hearing aid covers are sleeves that fit over the hearing aid body and protect them from dirt, moisture, sweat, etc. These covers come in different versions, however the most effective in my opinion are the stretchy, plastic types. These keep out the most moisture and don't stop the microphone from picking up crucial sound input.

Hearing Aid Boots (Shoes)

Hearing aid boots, sometimes called shoes, are additions to the hearing aid that either join onto or replace the battery door piece of the hearing aid with a small pin. The boot is most commonly used to accommodate FM systems, Bluetooth or other devices so that it can be used along with the hearing aid, especially if the HA is not equipped by itself. Many HA's have BT and FM integrated and don't require a boot, but they are still very popular.

CHAPTER 6

STORIES

Show and Tell

When I was in Kindergarten, I was the only one in my entire school with hearing aids. My parents were worried that I would feel different or left out from the rest of the students. We had a weekly show and tell morning in our class and most kids brought in their newest, best race car or action figure, but I decided to look everywhere in my house for my old pair of hearing aids (that we kept for backup). I eventually found them at the bottom of a drawer and went on a mission to get my favorite stuffed animal. This animal was none other than a Lamb named Lamby (of course). As I got ready for school, I was ready to proudly show off my Show and Tell item for the week to my parents before leaving the house for school. I put hearing aids on Lamby to show everyone that she has hearing aids too!

The point to this story is to not worry about your child too much, as they WILL learn to embrace it.

The Difference Between Hearing and Talking

Another day in school, I was having hearing aid troubles. I had gone to the teacher to tell her that I couldn't hear anything, but I was silently mouthing and acting out the words for her. This made the teacher nervous and I was sent down to the principal's office where the school proceeded to call my parents about how I suddenly couldn't hear or speak.

My father came flying into the school to see what happened and are talking to me trying to figure out the problem. When asked what the problem is, I mouthed "I can't hear" while pointing to my ears, my dad looked at me and said, "Okay, but that doesn't mean you can't talk!!"

Then, I tried talking and incredibly, I could!

The idea of this story is that children don't always get the
concepts that we do with experience, even if it's common
sense, which is intensified when something scary happens
like suddenly not being able to hear because of a hearing
aid problem which they mentally connect to something
similar such as another form of communication. Your child
will gain valuable experience every day that they go
through hearing loss, they will become knowledgeable
about the problems and situations that can arise, as well as
learn how to understand when a scary situation may be an
easy fix and doesn't come with everlasting consequences.

AFTERWORD

As hard as it is to accept that your child has a hearing disability and to navigate the challenges that come with it, with your help they will be absolutely fine. You've already taken a big step to getting ahead of this by educating yourself about hearing loss, specifically in children. Take time for yourself and your loved ones, understand what your child's challenges are and how to help towards conquering them. New research and technology comes out every single day that will help make hearing loss less debilitating. Your child will be able to have a perfectly successful, normal life during their childhood formative years, education, family life and beyond with hearing impairment.